Flu Therapy
A Natural and Herbal Approach

Elizabeth Wotton, N.D.

CONTENTS

Introduction

Each year, millions of people suffer from the influenza virus. Most recover in a matter of days, but many suffer complications that can lead to long-term problems — pneumonia, encephalitis, and even death. And while conventional medicine is effective at fighting the secondary bacterial infections that can accompany a viral illness, it has little to offer in the way of fighting the flu.

Fortunately, each of us has a built-in network of defense mechanisms that protects us against disease-causing viruses and other infectious microorganisms.

Herbs support this network in a variety of ways. Some herbs contain compounds that kill harmful microbes on contact or stimulate the immune system to increase the activity of white blood cells. Other herbs aid in a more indirect way — by thinning congestion-causing mucus to facilitate its excretion, by modulating a fever, or by enhancing resistance to infection. Still others can be used for comfort — to alleviate aches and pains, to soothe an upset stomach, or to help induce a more restful sleep.

While there may be times when we need to resort to over-the-counter medications or prescription pharmaceuticals, nature has provided us with a bountiful pharmacy that we can grow in our own backyards. Read on to find out everything you need to know about flu — and how herbs can help you prevent and treat it.

Danger Over the Counter

Reye's syndrome (RS) is a serious complication of certain viral infections, including the flu. Children under the age of 15 are most susceptible. Aspirin and other over-the-counter medications that contain salicylates increase a child's risk of RS. Typically occurring 3 to 5 days after a viral infection begins, RS causes persistent vomiting, lethargy, confusion, personality changes, convulsions, and loss of consciousness. Without early diagnosis and treatment, RS can cause brain damage and liver dysfunction. The best treatment is prevention: *Never give a child aspirin during a flu infection.* Other salicylate-containing medicines to avoid during the flu include Alka-Seltzer, Anacin, Bufferin, Dristan, Excedrin, and Pepto-Bismol.

Fall Means Flu

As the days become shorter and colder, the influenza virus starts warming up for its annual onslaught. For most of the Northern Hemisphere, autumn heralds not only the beginning of colder weather but also the start of flu season. In the months that follow, travelers crisscrossing the country, cooler temperatures, and increased levels of stress add up to conditions that are ideal for viruses to flourish.

Once viruses gain a foothold, they spread easily from person to person through respiratory droplets, those aerosol vapors that disperse through a sneeze or a cough. For susceptible people, the virus settles in quickly, bringing those familiar muscle aches, fevers, and chills that are the hallmark of the flu.

But the presence of viruses and other infectious organisms in your environment doesn't necessarily mean that you'll get sick. Developing a healthful lifestyle, taking precautions to minimize your risk of infection, and knowing how to prevent and manage the flu safely will help you stay healthy no matter what the season.

An Alphabet Soup of Viruses

There are numerous types of viral infections. Many infections commonly referred to as flu are not really caused by influenza viruses. In fact, there are only three identified influenza viruses: influenza type A, type B, and type C.

Types A and B are responsible for epidemics of respiratory illness and are associated with severe illness, complications, hospitalization, and death.

Type C is usually mild and may come and go without symptoms. It does not cause or contribute to epidemics, so it is not considered a serious health threat. That's why prevention and treatment efforts are targeted at only types A and B.

No One Is Immune to the Flu

In the United States, influenza virus infections are most prominent from November through April, peaking between late December and early March. Each year, between 10 and 40 million people in the United States get the flu. Flu outbreaks typically occur in small, localized populations, such as schools, daycare facilities, and families, and last for only short periods of time. And although most people will recover without complications or lingering effects, 1 percent will require hospitalization for severe illness. Of those 1 percent who are hospitalized, about 8 percent will die from complications directly caused by the flu.

Like some other viruses, the influenza virus gradually evolves over time so that the virus that was causing illness last year may return this year in an altered form. That's why no one is ever really immune to the flu. As "new" viruses, these mutated viruses initially go unrecognized by the immune system. And by the time the immune system has had a chance to respond, the virus is well established and spreading efficiently throughout the surrounding communities.

That's how epidemics, or localized outbreaks, start. Pandemics, or worldwide epidemics of influenza, occur when the structure of a flu virus changes suddenly and dramatically. It becomes sufficiently different from previous flu viruses so that large numbers of people have no immune protection against it. These influenza pandemics are rare but devastating. Although only three influenza pandemics have occurred in the past century, among them they caused more than 20 million deaths worldwide.

Although both influenza and SARS-CoV-2, the virus which causes the corona virus, have a strong affinity for the respiratory system, they are unrelated. SARS-CoV-2 (or COVID-19) is a novel virus, which means that we had no available treatments or immunity to the pathogen when it emerged in late 2019, whereas with influenza we have a long history of interacting with the virus.

Is It the Flu?

Influenza usually starts with a fever — generally 100 to 103°F (38–39°C) in adults, 102 to 105°F (39–40°C) in children. Respiratory symptoms, such as a runny or stuffy nose and cough, may appear suddenly, along with a sore throat, headache, muscle aches, and extreme fatigue. The fever phase of the flu typically lasts 3 to 4 days, followed by several days of continued weakness and fatigue. It is not uncommon for the fever to have a second peak following several days of a normal temperature. This may indicate a secondary bacterial infection, especially if accompanied by worsening symptoms. Flus complicated by bacterial infection may require antibiotic therapy. If you think you're suffering from a secondary infection, call your doctor for appropriate treatment.

Children are more likely to exhibit systemic symptoms, including nausea, vomiting, and diarrhea, when they have the flu. "Stomach flu" is simply a misnomer often used to describe gastrointestinal infections caused by other microorganisms.

The entire course of influenza usually lasts 1 to 2 weeks.

Flu or Cold?

Is it the flu or just a common cold? It's sometimes difficult to differentiate between the two. Here's a checklist of signs and symptoms characteristic of each.

	Flu	Cold
Fever	Over 100.5°F (38°C)	Slight or none
Muscle aches	Yes	None
Headache	Usually	Occasionally
Sore throat	Usually	Occasionally
Fatigue	Moderate to severe	None to moderate
Congestion	Sinus and/or chest	Sinus and/or chest

When Flu Gets Complicated

People over the age of 65 and those with chronic immune deficiency or disorders involving the respiratory or cardiovascular system may be at increased risk for developing serious illness and complications when they get the flu.

On average, approximately 20,000 Americans die from complications of influenza each year. These complications include pneumonia, encephalitis (inflammation of the brain), myocarditis (inflammation of the heart), and Reye's syndrome (brain and liver damage). It's important to remember that while most cases of influenza resolve on their own with time, the flu can be a serious illness, especially to the elderly, the very young, and those whose immune systems are already weakened by chronic conditions.

Who Should Take the Flu Vaccine?

The flu vaccine is an annual immunization designed to provide protection against those flu viruses projected to be most prevalent that season. The Centers for Disease Control and Prevention (CDC) recommends the vaccine for people who are at high risk of developing serious complications from influenza infections — those over the age of 65 and those with chronic immune deficiency or disorders that involve the respiratory or cardiovascular system. In addition, pregnant women, children who are at risk for Reye's syndrome (e.g., children on aspirin therapy), and those who are in frequent contact with high-risk patients (e.g., health practitioners, caretakers, and household members) should consider an annual flu shot.

CDC guidelines suggest that the flu vaccine be administered between September and mid-November for maximum protection during the flu season. Annual administration is necessary because of the changing nature of viruses and the temporary protection provided by the vaccine.

The vaccine is a concoction of dead influenza virus particles that are cultivated using hen's eggs. Serious side effects of the vaccine may occur in those who have allergies to eggs or other vaccine components. Other side effects include soreness at the injection site, headaches, and low-grade fever.

The effectiveness of the vaccine is limited by the fact that the influenza virus strains included in the vaccine are chosen 9 to 10 months before the influenza season begins. Mutating influenza viruses and incorrect guesses about which viruses will spread limit the usefulness of the vaccine. The CDC reports that in healthy young adults, the vaccine is 70 to 90 percent effective in preventing illness. However, healthy young adults are also the least likely to suffer a serious bout of the flu or its complications. The vaccine is most useful in elderly and debilitated populations where, though it is less effective, it may nonetheless reduce the severity of an illness and the likelihood of serious complications.

Big Medicine's Big Guns

The antiviral pharmaceuticals amantadine and rimantadine have been shown to be effective at interfering with the replication of the influenza A virus. By halting the virus's ability to reproduce, the antivirals give your immune system time to mobilize and take action against the infection. These drugs can be administered in prevention, before infection, and as treatment within the first 48 hours of illness. They may be used for people who are at high risk and who have not received the flu vaccine. Serious side effects associated with amantadine and rimantadine are alterations in central nervous system and gastrointestinal function, such as delirium, seizure, hallucination, and stomach upset.

Our Natural Defenses

Given the sometimes deadly nature of flu, it's fortunate that the body has a number of built-in defenses.

The surfaces of your body form a physical barrier with secretions, mucus, and oils that contain immune-promoting substances called immunoglobulins. These immunoglobulins, specifically secretory immunoglobulin A, are present on the skin, along the entire gastrointestinal tract, in sinus passages, and in the lungs. In addition, tiny hairs, called cilia, help trap foreign particles in the respiratory tract and assist in their removal. Fevers, increased mucus production, vomiting, and diarrhea are other ways in which the body immobilizes, kills, and eliminates infectious microbes.

The immune system also responds to a foreign intruder, such as a virus, by making an antibody that identifies the intruder and directs the body's defense. Each strain of virus requires a matching antibody. With many viruses, subsequent exposures do not necessarily lead to a recurrence of infection because of the ready-made antibodies at hand. This is illustrated by childhood diseases, such as measles, mumps, and rubella, in which an infection results in lifelong immunity. We don't get these infections a second time because our antibodies are armed and dangerous.

On the other hand, because viruses are adept at changing their features, some — such as the flu virus — can make your immune system think they're a brand-new virus, then slip past your body's defenses and infect you over and over again.

There are several factors that make you more susceptible to disease. Visitors from out of town may introduce different germs into the local environment. A drier, cooler climate along with household heating systems acts to dry mucous membranes and inhibit their natural ability to protect you. In addition, the change of seasons, the beginning of the school year, chronic physical or emotional stress, and a succession of holidays (with the accompanying stress of family and in-laws, late nights, and sugar overload) are all factors that can wear you down and weaken your immune system. Like other opportunistic infectious organisms, viruses have the ability to lie dormant during times of good health and surface when conditions are once again conducive to infection.

Flu Prevention

You can help prevent the flu by restoring balance to your body, building a strong immune system, and minimizing your risks. Here's what I mean.

Balance Your Body

Learn how to listen to your body, then pay attention to its cues. Overriding symptoms such as fatigue and low energy by repeatedly ignoring their message can become self-defeating when that nagging, run-down feeling turns into a full-blown infection. Knowing when to stop and reestablish balance is the first step in taking charge of your health.

Fight dehydration. Adequate hydration with plain water is a crucial element for every function of the body. In flu prevention, sufficient water intake keeps mucous membranes moist and healthy, enhancing their natural resistance to harmful organisms. Unfortunately, the change of seasons, particularly autumn to winter, poses its own challenges. Cooler temperatures often mean lower humidity. Heating systems, especially wood-burning stoves, further dry the environment, leaving respiratory passages parched and less resistant to infection. That's why

---

How Well Do You Listen to Your Body?

Do you get sick more than two or three times a year?

Do you feel run-down or unwell more than one day a week or three days a month?

Do you feel better on the weekends and then begin to feel run-down again during the week?

Do you feel rested after a full night's sleep?

Are you often tired during the day?

Do you push yourself through the day?

Do you find yourself feeling irritable or snapping for no particular reason?

Take time to consider these questions. If you answered yes to more than three of them, you may need to listen more closely to the messages your body is sending you.

you need to drink even more water in the winter than the rest of the year. (*Hint:* Nosebleeds and dry, cracking skin are two signs that you need to drink more water.)

Forget packaged foods, caffeine, and sugars. To help create optimal health, begin by decreasing your intake of refined and processed foods. Limit your intake of sugar, baked goods (e.g., doughnuts, bagels, and cookies), pasta, bread, prepared foods, and any food that comes in a package. Avoid stimulants (e.g., caffeine), alcohol, sodas, and simple sugars, including cane sugar, corn syrup, beet sugar, honey, maple syrup, fruit juice, and dried fruit. While you may receive short-term gain from the transient comfort of these foods, your body pays a long-term price. Refined and processed foods increase the body's excretion of important vitamins and minerals, such as B vitamins and magnesium, which are required for a healthy immune system.

Shop organically. Learn to listen to your body's needs. When you do, you'll find that rather than filling up on empty calories, your body wants to be replenished with wholesome, nutritious foods. Pesticides, hormones, and additives present in our food supply place a heavy burden on the body. If you eat foods contaminated with these substances, your body wastes energy and resources detoxifying itself instead of gaining strength. That's why you make a commitment to buy organically grown or raised produce, poultry, and meats.

Eat mindfully. How you eat is every bit as important as what you eat. Take time to create and enjoy your meals. Give yourself the space to appreciate the food that you're taking in for sustenance. Remember that digestion begins in the mouth. Breathe between bites and chew your food thoroughly. Cultivating awareness by allowing yourself to experience the present moment will guide you to a more healthful way of eating.

Build a Strong Immune System

The immune system, with its multiple facets, has specific requirements for nourishing and restoring itself. Good nutrition, moderate exercise, effective stress-coping strategies, and healthy relationships are key factors in keeping it on an even keel and ready to respond to trouble. The following tips will help you give your immune system what it needs to defend your body against the flu.

Load up on foods rich in vitamin A and carotenes. Vitamin A (retinol) and carotenes protect against infection by maintaining the integrity of mucous membranes. Vitamin A is found primarily in animal sources (e.g., beef, chicken, and dairy products), while carotenes are found in brightly colored vegetables (e.g., carrots and yams) and dark leafy greens.

Replenish vitamin C. Vitamin C (ascorbic acid) optimizes immune function and protects cells from damage caused by inflammation, a side effect of infection and your immune system's fight against it. Because ascorbic acid is a water-soluble vitamin, it is not stored in the body and needs to be continually replenished. Foods high in vitamin C include orange juice, peppers, grapefruit, broccoli, strawberries, and mango.

Maintain your zinc reserves. Zinc is the second most abundant trace mineral in the body, after iron. It lowers the incidence of illness, improves immune function, and speeds recovery. Zinc is found mainly in animal products, especially red meat, oysters, and other shellfish. Legumes (e.g., lima beans, soybeans, and pinto beans), whole grains, and pumpkin seeds also contain high amounts of zinc, though other compounds in these foods may inhibit its absorption.

Get adequate amounts of essential fatty acids. Essential fatty acids (omega-3 and omega-6 fats) have a regulatory effect on the immune system and are a necessary component of enhancing the strength of the body's tissues. These fats are found in nuts (e.g., walnuts, almonds, and hazelnuts), seeds (e.g., sesame, pumpkin, and flax), and cold-water fish (e.g., salmon, mackerel, and sardines).

Get on your feet. Exercising 30 to 60 minutes three or four times a week has a strengthening effect on the immune system, making it more resilient and able to withstand adverse conditions. If you suffer from chronic illness or have a circulatory-related condition, be sure to have your exercise regimen approved by your healthcare provider.

Zap stress. Learning to view stress as a challenge and meeting it head-on is an empowering experience that may actually enhance your well-being. Emotions are directly tied to immune function. Feelings of hopelessness and despair inhibit the ability of the immune system to respond appropriately to challenges. Relaxation techniques, meditation, yoga, exercise, journaling, and biofeedback are just some of the numerous ways to effectively manage stress.

Build nurturing relationships. Healthy relationships based on mutual respect and understanding — and that allow free communication — are essential to well-being. The benefits of relationships come not just from giving of oneself but from receiving as well. Too often we isolate ourselves rather than reach out for support. Take time to develop a network among your family, friends, and community. Seek relationships that nurture and sustain you in all aspects of your life.

Quiet mind and body. Setting aside time every day for meditation or prayer quiets the mind and relaxes the body, allowing for greater integration of body, mind, and spirit and an increased sense of well-being. Studies have shown that the relaxation response induced by a meditative state is a powerful enhancer of immune function.

Minimize Your Risk

Chances are good that no matter how careful you are, you'll encounter someone with the flu every fall. And while it's impossible to avoid all challenges and stress, here are a few simple steps you can take to beat the odds of getting sick.

Sleep. Consistently restful sleep is essential to maintaining good health. Your immune system does its best work when it is well rested. Catching up on your sleep on the weekends may feel good temporarily, but it can't make up for the effects of dragging your exhausted self through the workweek. Chronic sleep deprivation compromises immune function and makes us more susceptible to illness.

Travel only when necessary. Traveling long-distance may contribute to illness in two ways: by mingling germs from two separate and distant locales and by requiring you to spend time in a confined space, often with many people. Airplane travel provides ideal conditions for the exchange of diseases: dry, recirculated air; crowded conditions; and, for many passengers, a stressful situation.

Wash your hands frequently. We are constantly exchanging germs with other people and the environment we share. One of the primary ways we do it is with our hands. Opening doors, turning on water faucets in public rest rooms, covering our mouths to sneeze or cough, blowing our noses, shaking hands, sharing pens, pushing elevator buttons, gripping escalator railings, and holding phones are only a few ways in which we acquire and transmit germs to and from our surroundings. That's why you should make a point of washing your hands several times during the day and, especially, on returning home. Not only will you protect yourself from the germs that others have left behind, but you also will minimize the chances of spreading your own germs to others.

A Commonsense Approach to Treating the Flu

Even the healthiest, least stressed people occasionally succumb to the flu — and there's nothing to do but surrender to the process, cancel the week's schedule, then support your body's work with rest, nutrition, and herbs. Here's how to get back on your feet.

Eat simply. Eliminate dairy products, including milk, cheese, and ice cream. Dairy encourages the formation of mucus and promotes congestion. Avoid foods with lots of protein — meat, for example — which require a lot of energy to digest. Favor soups and broths, as well as steamed vegetables and cooked grains, such as oatmeal, barley, millet, and rice.

Sip and slurp. Frequent sips of tea, diluted juice (fruit or vegetable), soups, and water throughout the day will help maintain the fluids, minerals, and electrolytes you need to get well.

Let your fever work for you. A fever is one of your body's best defenses. Do not reduce a healthy fever with over-the-counter medications, such as Tylenol, unless the fever becomes dangerously high or you're very uncomfortable. (See the box below for tips on supporting a healthy fever.) Applying cool, damp cloths to the forehead and chest is a safe way to relieve the discomfort of a fever.

Natural Fever Aids

Fevers are your body's attempt to immobilize or kill harmful organisms. Children tend to have higher temperatures than adults without any adverse effects.

- **For fevers of 101°F (38°C) or less:** Increase fluids, including water, diluted juices, and herbal teas, to avoid becoming dehydrated. Drink herbal teas to support a healthy fever. These warm fluids warm the body, augmenting the infection-fighting increase in temperature, and stimulate perspiration to prevent too high a fever.
- **For persistent fevers (those that last 3 to 4 days) of 101°F (38°C) or higher:** In addition to the above, include herbs such as elder, peppermint, and yarrow to promote perspiration and cool the body. Lower the fever with tepid baths and compresses using cooled herbal infusions.

Rest, rest, rest! Stay in bed, sleep as much as you like, and avoid any unnecessary activities.

Avoid drastic temperature changes and becoming chilled. Stay warm and change into dry clothes after fever-induced sweats. A hot-water bottle wrapped in flannel and held close to the body can help ease feverish chills.

Supplement your immune system. Although it's important to include dietary sources of immune-enhancing nutrients while you have the flu, it's also important to take additional vitamin and mineral supplements. *Caution:* Pregnant women should consult a physician before taking supplements.

- *Vitamin A:* 10,000 IU one or two times daily for adults; 5,000 IU daily for children. Mixed carotenes or beta-carotenes may be taken instead of vitamin A and at higher doses (25,000 IU per day for adults; 10,000 IU daily for children).

- *Vitamin C:* 1,000 mg two or three times daily for adults; 250 to 500 mg two or three times daily for children. Take a buffered form of vitamin C to avoid stomach upset with high doses.

- *Zinc:* 15 mg one or two times daily for adults; 10 mg daily for children. Zinc lozenges are especially beneficial with sore throats. Take commercial preparations as directed.

- *Essential fatty acids:* 1,000 to 1,500 mg one or two times daily for adults. Alternatively, take 1 tablespoon of flaxseed oil one or two times daily; children can take ½ to 1 teaspoon daily. Essential fatty acids are fragile and need to be stored in dark containers and in a cool place. The beneficial effects of the oil are destroyed by light and heat.

When to Seek Help

Fevers over 103°F (39°C) that do not respond to fever-reducing treatments, severe vomiting, and severe diarrhea require immediate medical attention. Losing fluids through feverish sweats, vomiting, and diarrhea may cause serious dehydration or metabolic imbalances, particularly in the elderly and young children. A child with a high fever may even experience convulsions, become confused, or lose consciousness. Symptoms that are not improving or are worsening after 3 or 4 days of treatment may indicate severe illness or complications. If any of these signs or symptoms occur, consult your healthcare provider immediately or call 911 for emergency medical assistance.

Twelve Herbs to Beat the Flu

Herbs are a gentle and effective way to support your body during the flu season. They strengthen the body's resistance to disease and promote its natural defenses. In treating the flu, herbs can stimulate the immune system, aid in eliminating the virus, and alleviate discomfort all at the same time. They address every facet of the infection. The ground rules for using herbs are these:

- Gentle herbs in teas and glycerites should be used for children and for mild infections (those with low fever and few symptoms). More serious infections (characterized by high fever, sore throat, cough, aches and pains, fatigue, diarrhea, and so on) require higher doses at more frequent intervals.
- If the symptoms do not abate or are worsening 3 or 4 days after you initiate herbal treatment, check with your doctor.
- Those at high risk for complications — people over the age of 65 and those with chronic immune deficiency or disorders involving the respiratory or cardiovascular system — should seek medical attention whenever serious infections threaten and use herbs as a complement to conventional therapy.

A Glossary of Medicinal Herb Terms

Analgesic: Provides pain relief when taken internally

Anodyne: Provides pain relief when applied topically

Anticatarrhal: Inhibits the production of mucus and assists in resolving congestion

Antimicrobial: Inhibits or kills bacteria, viruses, and other microorganisms

Antiseptic: Inhibits the growth of microorganisms

Antispasmodic: Releases tension and spasm; relieves cramping

Antiviral: Directly inhibits or kills viruses

Astringent: Tones and tightens tissues, making them more resistant to infection

A Quick Guide to Quick Relief

Some herbs work better than others for relieving particular symptoms of the flu. In the lists below, herbs appropriate for treating particular symptoms or boosting particular systems are given in order of strength. The last herb in each category is no less effective than the first but should be used when a more gentle effect is desired, such as when treating children. See the individual herb listings beginning on page 16 for specific information on dosage and preparation.

Cough: Elder, licorice, garlic, ginger, cleavers

Fatigue: Chamomile, lemon balm, catnip

Fever: Yarrow, ginger, elder, garlic, mint, lemon balm, catnip

Immune support: Echinacea, licorice, garlic, ginger, lemon balm, elder, cleavers

Muscle aches: Ginger, chamomile, lemon balm, catnip

Nausea: Ginger, peppermint, chamomile, lemon balm, catnip

Sinus congestion: Garlic, ginger, eyebright, peppermint, yarrow, elder

Sore throat: Licorice, ginger, garlic, chamomile, eyebright, yarrow

---

Carminative: Relaxes the stomach and relieves spasm in the intestinal tract

Demulcent: Soothes inflamed, irritated mucous membranes

Diaphoretic: Promotes perspiration; assists the body in eliminating toxins

Expectorant: Aids in expelling mucus from the chest and throat

Immune stimulant: Increases the activity of specific immune functions

Lymphatic: Stimulates lymph circulation; aids in the elimination of toxins and products of inflammation

Mucolytic: Breaks up, thins, and resolves mucus

Nervine: Soothes nervous tension and encourages relaxation without sedation

Sedative: Decreases pain and nervous irritability by inhibiting central nervous system function

Catnip (Nepeta cataria)

Parts used: Whole herb
Actions: Antispasmodic, carminative, diaphoretic, mild sedative
Medicinal uses: Although this herb is well known for its stimulating effect on cats, it actually has a sedating effect on humans. Catnip is an excellent remedy for children, as it calms an upset stomach, alleviates diarrhea, quiets restlessness, induces sleep, and gently breaks a fever by encouraging perspiration.
Dosage: Adults should take 1 cup of catnip tea three or four times daily. Children should take ¼ to ½ cup of tea three or four times daily.

Chamomile (Matricaria recutita)

Parts used: Flowers
Actions: Anodyne, antimicrobial, antiseptic, carminative, mucolytic, nervine
Medicinal uses: Chamomile is a gentle but powerful herb, especially beneficial for children. Its uses for calming and inducing sleep are well known, as it is typically included in commercial sleep-promoting preparations. Chamomile also calms digestive upset by relieving diarrhea, nausea, and cramping. Its antimicrobial compounds and mucus-thinning action help resolve congestion while reducing infection. When taken orally in teas or tinctures, chamomile soothes a sore throat and cools inflamed tissues.
Dosage: Adults should take 1 cup of chamomile tea three or four times daily. Children should take ¼ to ½ cup of tea three or four times daily.
Caution: Chamomile may occasionally induce an allergic reaction in individuals with hay fever and allergies to ragweed.

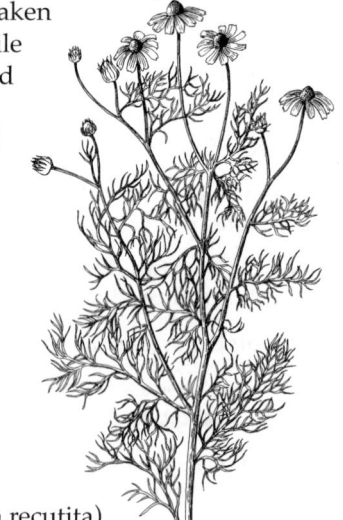

Chamomile (Matricaria recutita)

Cleavers (Galium aparine)

Parts used: Whole herb
Actions: Astringent, demulcent, lymphatic
Medicinal uses: Cleavers helps support the immune system by stimulating lymph circulation and encouraging drainage from swollen lymph nodes. Its demulcent and astringent properties make it a powerful ally in treating respiratory infections, as it both soothes and tones tissues. Use the fresh herb whenever possible; the drying process destroys many of cleavers's beneficial compounds. Cleavers is abundant in spring, growing in shady, moist ground. It's an excellent herb to include in spring tonics.
Dosage: Adults should take 1 cup of cleavers tea two times daily. Children should take ¼ to ½ cup of tea two times daily.

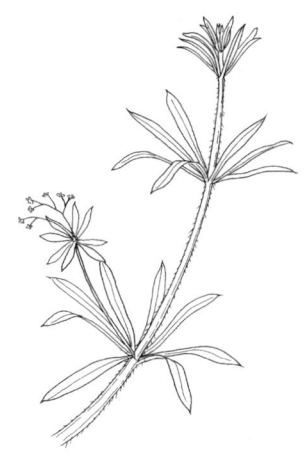

Cleavers (Galium aparine)

Echinacea (Echinacea *spp.*)

Parts used: Whole herb of *E. angustifolia;* whole herb and root of *E. purpurea;* whole herb and root of *E. pallida.*
Actions: Antimicrobial, antiseptic, antiviral, immune stimulant
Medicinal uses: Long used by Native Americans as a remedy for infections, fevers, and snakebites, echinacea was adopted by early American healers as a "cure-all" and tonic for any ailment. Echinacea is currently one of the most researched herbs in botanical medicine, and its historical uses have been shown to be well founded. All varieties have been shown to be effective in stimulating immune system activity. Its antiviral properties and immune-enhancing compounds make it ideal for treating influenza. It is not necessary to use standardized extracts to achieve medicinal effects, as many of echinacea's beneficial compounds are readily available in teas, tinctures, and the fresh juice. One side effect of taking echinacea orally is a tingling and numb sensation in the mouth. While this may be an annoyance, it can also provide temporary relief to a sore throat.
Dosage: Adults should take 1 cup of echinacea tea or 30 to 60 drops of echinacea tincture three or four times daily. Children should take ¼ to ½ cup of tea or 10 to 20 drops of tincture three or four times daily.

Elder (Sambucus nigra)

Parts used: Flowers and berries
Actions: Anticatarrhal, antiviral, diaphoretic, immune stimulant
Medicinal uses: Elder is often found planted at the entrance to gardens for protection — a carryover from the old superstitious belief that elder warded off evil spirits and witches. Elder has traditionally been used as a respiratory tonic and aids in relieving congestion. It provides good overall support for the flu, especially when it's accompanied by a sore throat and fever. The herb soothes the mucous membranes and helps reduce inflammation throughout the respiratory tract. (See the box below for instructions on making an elderberry cough medicine.)
Dosage: Adults should take 1 cup of elder tea three times daily. Children should take ¼ to ½ cup of tea two or three times daily.

Elderberry Syrup: A Natural Cough Medicine

Elderberries picked in late summer or early fall can easily be made into a syrup and used alone or as a base for other cough remedies. Place 1 cup of elderberries in a clean jar. Add 16 ounces of apple cider vinegar and let steep 12 hours or overnight. Strain and place in a nonreactive pot. Add 2 cups of raw sugar and simmer for 20 minutes, until sugar is melted. Store in a clean, dark jar in the refrigerator.

Eyebright (Euphrasia officinalis)

Parts used: Whole herb
Actions: Anticatarrhal, anti-inflammatory, astringent
Medicinal uses: Eyebright is a gentle astringent that helps reduce excessive mucus secretions and relieve irritated respiratory passages. It's particularly indicated when there is eye pain and sensitivity to light from fevers or the flu. Use eyebright when symptoms are concentrated in the head with sinus tenderness, eye pain, and copious drainage. This plant is threatened in the wild, so look for cultivated eyebright.
Dosage: Adults should take 1 cup of eyebright tea two or three times daily. Children should take ¼ to ½ cup of eyebright tea two or three times daily.

Garlic (Allium sativum)

Part used: Bulb
Actions: Antiseptic, antispasmodic, antiviral, diaphoretic, expectorant, mucolytic
Medicinal uses: Anyone who has eaten raw garlic knows that it contains pungent substances that remain detectable in the breath for hours afterward. These aromatic compounds contain the antibacterial and antiviral properties that make garlic an ideal herb for fighting the flu. Garlic has a rich history of acclaim for everything from fighting disease to warding off vampires. In 1721, when the French city of Marseilles was overrun with the plague, the four condemned criminals who were recruited as grave diggers were found to be immune to the disease. Their secret was a brew of macerated garlic in wine. This "four thieves' vinegar"

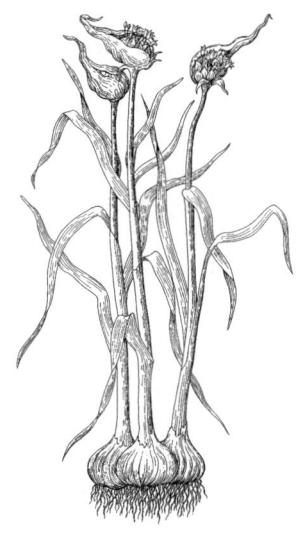

Garlic (Allium sativum)

is still widely available in France today. Garlic has enjoyed widespread medicinal use; however, only raw garlic has had documented beneficial effects.
Dosage: Adults should take 1 cup of garlic tea three times daily. Children should take ¼ to ½ cup of garlic tea two or three times daily. Also, make an effort to include raw garlic in your diet.

Ginger (Zingiber officinale)

Part used: Rhizome
Actions: Anti-inflammatory, antispasmodic, antiviral, carminative, diaphoretic
Medicinal uses: Ginger has both stimulating and relaxing properties. It encourages circulation, which helps increase perspiration and relieve a fever while maintaining a feeling of warmth and calm in the body. Small sips of ginger tea stimulate the release of digestive enzymes and alleviate nausea and spasm. Ginger encourages blood flow to the head and chest, which helps deliver its antiviral compounds to those areas while aiding in the drainage of congestion. Its anti-inflammatory actions also help relieve muscle aches and pain.
Dosage: Adults should take 1 cup of ginger tea three or four times daily. Children should take ¼ to ½ cup of tea three or four times daily.

Lemon Balm (Melissa officinalis)

Parts used: Whole herb
Actions: Antispasmodic, antiviral, carminative, nervine
Medicinal uses: Lemon balm's citrus-scented volatile oil is responsible for most of the herb's medicinal actions. Taken orally as tea or tincture, lemon balm eases tension, calms the mind, stimulates digestion, and reduces a fever. Inhaled in steams, the volatile oil supports the respiratory tract with its antiviral properties. Its pleasant fragrance elevates mood and both calms and energizes the mind.
Dosage: Adults should take 1 cup of lemon balm tea three or four times daily. Children should take ¼ to ½ cup of tea three or four times daily.
Caution: Lemon balm is a mild inhibitor of thyroid-stimulating hormone. If you have a sluggish thyroid or are taking thyroid medication, check with your doctor before using this herb.

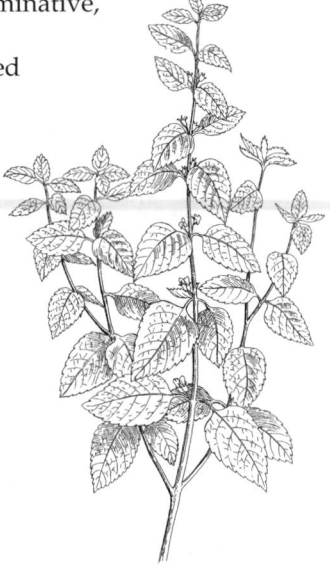

Lemon balm
(Melissa officinalis)

Licorice (Glycyrrhiza glabra)

Part used: Root
Actions: Anti-inflammatory, antiviral, demulcent, expectorant, immune stimulant
Medicinal uses: Licorice is an old folk remedy for coughs and digestive complaints. Current research has confirmed its antiviral and anti-inflammatory benefits, as well as the fact that it stimulates the immune system. Licorice helps increase the productivity of coughs, both releasing spasms and increasing the removal of mucus. It is an excellent herb for treating influenza because it both inhibits the replication of viruses and activates the immune system. Its sweet, pleasant taste makes licorice a good herb to use in combinations that include less palatable herbs.

Dosage: Adults should take 1 cup of licorice tea two or three times daily. Children should take ¼ to ½ cup of tea two or three times daily. *Caution:* Licorice root should not be used by those who have high blood pressure.

Peppermint (Mentha piperita)

Parts used: Whole herb
Actions: Antiseptic, analgesic, carminative, diaphoretic, nervine
Medicinal uses: Once used to crown Greeks and Romans on feast days, peppermint is a warming antispasmodic that relieves everything from fever to nausea. Its nervine properties aid in sleeplessness and restlessness. It can be used alone or as a taste enhancer in other tea or tincture formulas. The volatile peppermint oil released when its leaves are crushed or simmered in steaming teas kills germs in the respiratory tract and alleviates congestion. Used topically, the oil encourages circulation, bringing soothing warmth to the affected area.
Dosage: Adults should take 1 cup of peppermint tea three or four times daily. Children should take ¼ to ½ cup of peppermint tea three or four times daily.

Yarrow (Achillea millefolium)

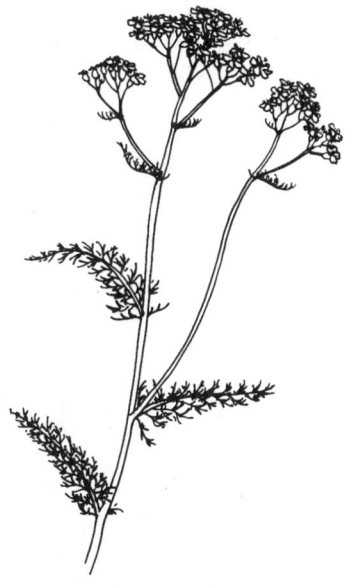

Parts used: Flowers or whole herb
Actions: Anti-inflammatory, astringent, diaphoretic
Medicinal uses: Drinking hot yarrow tea induces moderate perspiration and helps lower a fever. The tea's bitter taste stimulates digestion and appetite and contributes to its usefulness as an overall tonic for malaise and debility.
Dosage: Adults should take 1 cup of yarrow tea two or three times daily. Children should take ¼ to ½ cup of yarrow tea two or three times daily.

Yarrow (Achillea millefolium)

Herbal Medicine for Children

When you're feeling under the weather, the last thing you want is a foul-tasting brew. Children, especially, will resist icky-tasting medicine. On the other hand, they often like tastes and flavors that adults don't. When choosing a combination of herbs for your child, be sure to include some of the more pleasant-tasting herbs to offset any of the less palatable ones. If you should sample the formula in front of your child, be careful not to make a face of distaste. You can be sure that if your child senses that you don't like it, then he or she won't either.

Herbs can be mixed with juice or with other flavoring herbs to improve taste. Glycerite preparations are sweet and generally liked by children. If your child is having difficulty taking herbs orally, you can use other methods of administration, such as steams, baths, compresses, and rubs. The skin is highly absorbent, even more so in children, and is a wonderful way to introduce medicines into the system. Using an external application to provide herbal support is also a nice way to soothe a child who is restless and uncomfortable.

Herbal Dosages for Children

A rough gauge of a child's dose is to divide the adult dose in half. However, most herbalists use the following guideline:

$$\frac{\text{Age in years}}{\text{Age} + 12} = \text{portion of adult dose}$$

Example for a 4-year-old:

$$\frac{4}{4 + 12} = \text{\textonequarter}_{16} = \text{one-fourth of the adult dose}$$

Using Herbs to Feel Better Fast

Herbs may be taken in a variety of ways to suit a variety of purposes. As food, teas, and tinctures or glycerite preparations, herbs assert a direct effect on the digestive tract. Many of them have an affinity for specific tissues, which makes them useful in directing medicinal activity and synergistic herbs to a localized area. Others have systemic effects, tonifying and cleansing the body or helping relieve exhaustion and debility.

How to Use Herbs Safely

The herbs discussed here are generally considered to be mild and safe for use by both children and adults. But any substance that we ingest or apply topically has the potential for an unwelcome side effect. While the known effects are listed in "Twelve Herbs to Beat the Flu" (beginning on page 14), our individual biochemistry is unique and always leaves the door open to the unexpected. So pay attention to your body's response and discontinue any herb you suspect of causing an adverse effect.

Adverse reactions or sensitivities to herbs often present themselves with a headache or nausea. If you experience either of these conditions or symptoms, consult an experienced herbalist or health practitioner for guidance.

In baths and steams, herbs release volatile oils that are natural antiseptics and act on respiratory passages. The fragrance of these oils has a secondary effect on the emotional centers of the brain, inducing a feeling of calm and helping relieve discomfort. And applying an herbal preparation directly to the skin as a compress or rub initiates an immediate localized response, with gradual systemic effects.

It's best to employ more than one herb to provide relief for different symptoms and overall immune support. For example, if a child has a fever with nausea and restlessness, you may want to combine yarrow (to support the fever), ginger (to ease the nausea), catnip (to calm the restlessness), and echinacea (to support the immune system).

In general, alcohol-based tinctures are stronger than teas and glycerites because alcohol extracts a broader spectrum of herbal compounds. This is not always true, however, as many herbs have beneficial properties that are extracted in water or glycerine.

Making and Using Herbal Teas

There are two ways to prepare herbal tea. You can make an infusion, in which the herb is steeped, or you can make a decoction, in which the plant matter is simmered over time.

Infusions. To extract medicinal properties from leaves, flowers, berries, or seeds, you'll want to infuse them. Pour 1 cup of boiling water over 1 heaping teaspoon of dried herbs or 2 tablespoons of fresh herbs. (If you're using berries or seeds, crush them first.) Cover, let steep 10 to 15 minutes, strain, and drink.

> ## What's "Herb"?
>
> *Herb* means the aerial parts of a plant — not just the leaves but all of the plant that grows above ground.

Decoctions. Decoctions are made by simmering root, bark, and other woody parts of the plant to extract their medicinal properties. Add 1 heaping teaspoon of dried root to 1 cup of water. Cover, bring to a boil, then simmer 15 to 20 minutes. Strain the herbs and enjoy.

Combinations. When you're making a tea with both roots and leaves, you'll both infuse and decoct: Simmer the roots 20 minutes, remove from the heat, add the leaves and stir, then cover and steep 10 to 20 minutes longer.

SORE THROAT SOOTHER

Sip this warming tea to relieve a sore throat.

    1 part chamomile flowers
    1 part eyebright herb
    1 part gingerroot
      Honey

Decoct the gingerroot for 10 minutes, then remove from heat. Add the eyebright and chamomile, cover, and steep 10 minutes. Drink warm, sweetened with honey if desired. Adults can take 1 cup four to six times a day; children can take ¼ to ½ cup three or four times a day.

Herb Pops Soothe a Sore Throat

Herbal ice pops are a good way to relieve a sore throat and introduce fluids. Dilute grape or apple juice by half with a cooled medicinal tea made from one of the above recipes or from your own herbal repertory. Pour into trays for making ice pops and freeze.

IMMUNE BOOSTER TEA

This tea provides gentle yet effective support for the immune system.

> 2 **parts licorice root**
> 1 **part echinacea herb**
> 1 **part echinacea root**
> 1 **part garlic bulb**
> 1 **part ginger root**

Combine all ingredients. Decoct 20 minutes and drink warm. Adults can take 1 cup four to six times a day; children can take ¼ to ½ cup three or four times a day.

FEVER TEA

Use this tea to encourage perspiration during the fever phase of the flu. You may add a small amount of honey to offset the bitter taste of yarrow and make the tea more palatable. This combination can also be used for baths, steams, and compresses.

> 2 **parts elder flowers**
> 2 **parts yarrow flowers**
> 1 **part gingerroot**
> 1 **part peppermint herb**

Decoct the gingerroot for 10 minutes. Remove from heat, add the remaining ingredients, cover, and steep 10 minutes. Drink warm. Adults can take 1 cup four to six times a day; children can take ¼ to ½ cup three or four times a day.

CALMING TEA

This is an excellent tea for relieving restlessness and irritability, especially in children. The tea has a minty lemon flavor that most children enjoy.

> 2 **parts catnip herb**
> 2 **parts lemon balm herb**
> 1 **part chamomile flowers**
> 1 **part peppermint herb**

Combine all ingredients and infuse, covered, for 10 minutes. Drink warm. Adults can take 1 cup four to six times a day; children can take ¼ to ½ cup three or four times a day. Breathing in the vapors from the tea while sipping will help clear congested sinuses.

Tinctures and Glycerites

Tinctures are alcoholic extracts of herbs. They often have a sharp, unpleasant taste, but they are extremely potent. They may be added to hot water to dissipate the alcohol before ingesting. Glycerites are nonalcoholic extracts of herbs. They are generally sweet and more palatable to children. Tinctures and glycerites are available at most herb shops and natural foods stores. Tinctures should be stored in a cool, dark location, where they will keep for up to 2 years. Glycerites should be stored in the refrigerator, where they will keep for up to 3 months.

General dosages for tinctures and glycerites are as follows.

- **Tinctures for adults:** 30 to 60 drops two to four times daily
- **Tinctures for children:** 10 to 20 drops two to four times daily
- **Glycerites for adults:** 1 teaspoon three or four times daily
- **Glycerites for children:** ½ teaspoon three or four times daily

GINGER-GARLIC SYRUP BASE FOR TINCTURES

This is a good-tasting syrup that can be used alone or as a base for tinctures or other preparations.

> 1 **head of garlic**
> 1 **2-inch section of raw gingerroot**
> **Raw sugar (or substitute white sugar, brown sugar, or pasteurized honey)**

Peel and slice the garlic and the gingerroot. Layer in a clean glass jar and cover completely with sugar. Store in a cool, dark location for 3 days. Shake once or twice daily. (If you are using honey, you will need to repeat this process for an additional 4 days, for a total of 7 days.) Strain the syrup and store in the refrigerator, where it will keep for up to 3 months. Use as an immune-supporting syrup, to mix with tinctures to improve their taste, or as a base for other syrups.

HERBAL COUGH SYRUP

This formula contains potent antiviral herbs that boost immunity and strengthen the lungs. It is especially helpful in addressing persistent coughs and respiratory infections that settle in the chest.

> 2 ounces ginger-garlic syrup (see recipe on page 26)
> ½ ounce catnip tincture
> ½ ounce echinacea tincture
> ½ ounce elder flower tincture
> ½ ounce licorice root tincture

Mix all ingredients. Store in a dark glass container in a cool, dark location, where the syrup will keep for up to 1 year. Adults can take 60 to 90 drops three or four times daily; children can take 30 to 40 drops three or four times daily.

CHILDREN'S DECONGESTANT AND COUGH SYRUP

A gentle, effective cough remedy for children, this syrup can ease a cough while fighting infection and sinus congestion.

> 2 ounces elderberry syrup (see recipe on page 18)
> 1 ounce ginger-garlic syrup (see recipe on page 26)
> 1 ounce licorice root tincture
> 1 ounce peppermint tincture

Combine all ingredients. Store in a dark glass container in a cool, dark location, where the syrup will keep for up to 1 year. Children should take ½ teaspoon four to six times daily for coughs and congestion.

SINUS RELIEF

This formula helps clear sinus passages, protect the lungs, and boost immune function.

> 1 part cleavers tincture
> 1 part echinacea tincture
> 1 part elderberry syrup (see recipe on page 18)
> 1 part eyebright tincture
> 1 part gingerroot tincture

Combine all ingredients. Store in a dark glass container in a cool, dark location, where the syrup will keep for up to 1 year. Adults can take 60 to 90 drops three or four times daily; children can take 20 to 30 drops three or four times daily. To maximize the actions of the herbs, place the dosage in a cup of hot water and sip slowly.

COMFORT COMPOUND

This is an excellent remedy for muscle aches with general discomfort and restlessness.

> **2 parts chamomile tincture**
> **2 parts gingerroot tincture**
> **1 part lemon balm tincture**
> **1 part licorice root tincture**

Combine all ingredients. Store in a glass container in a cool, dark location, where it will keep for up to 2 years. Adults can take 60 to 90 drops three or four times daily; children can take 20 to 30 drops three or four times daily.

FLU FORMULA

Begin taking this formula at the first sign of the flu.

> **1 part echinacea tincture**
> **1 part elder tincture**
> **1 part eyebright tincture**
> **1 part gingerroot tincture**
> **1 part lemon balm tincture**
> **1 part licorice root tincture**

Combine all ingredients. Store in a cool, dark location, where it will keep for up to 2 years. Adults can take 60 to 90 drops every three to four hours. Children can take 20 to 30 drops three times daily.

Using Essential Oils

Fragrant herbs contain essential (volatile) oils that are antiseptic in nature. The oils can be used and applied in several ways. Inhaling their vapor in baths and steams helps fight infection in the respiratory passages. Combining the essential oil with a base oil and applying it to the skin aids in muscle aches and helps provide a localized heating effect that increases circulation and the delivery of nutrients to the area. It also transports waste products away from the site.

Caution: Do not take essential oils internally without the guidance of a qualified herbalist or healthcare practitioner.

AN HERBAL STEAM

This is an effective method for clearing congestion.

1 quart water
6–8 drops essential oil of chamomile, lemon balm, or peppermint

Heat the water on the stove. Remove from heat and add the herbal tincture. Using a large bath towel as a tent, lean over the pot and inhale the steam. Avoid becoming over-heated or getting your face too close to the hot steam. Blow your nose fre-quently to help ease congestion and clear the nasal passages for the healing vapors.

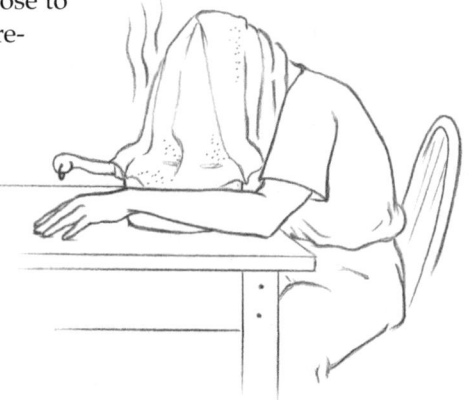

Tent a towel over both your head and the bowl to capture the aromatic steam.

An Herbal Bath

A therapeutic bath can be used at the first sign of flu or during the recovery phase, to relieve muscle pain and promote relax-ation. Soak in a hot bath for 10 minutes or until you begin to perspire. Get out of the tub slowly, dress warmly, and go imme-diately to bed. Be sure to drink copious fluids before, during, and after the bath to replenish the fluid lost from perspiration. Sipping a cup of hot ginger or yarrow tea while in the tub will enhance the warming effects of the water.

To ease aching muscles and encourage perspiration, add 1 quart of an herbal infusion of ginger, lemon balm, or pepper-mint to the bathwater. The fragrance will soothe, and the volatile oils will warm and relieve aching muscles.

Caution: Avoid hot baths when a fever over 100.5°F (38°C) is present. Hot baths are not advised for young children or the el-derly, who may be at risk for dehydration.

AN HERBAL RUB

These warming essential oils help increase circulation and relieve congestion.

Peppermint or lemon balm essential oil
Olive or almond oil

Combine the ingredients, using 20 drops of essential oil per 2 ounces of food-grade oil. Gently rub onto the sinus area or chest. This treatment is best done when you can spend 15 to 20 minutes lying down with your eyes closed. To enhance the heating effects of the oil when it's used on your chest, cover the rubbed area with a clean cloth, then place a hot-water bottle on top.

Caution: Use caution when applying the oil to your sinuses, as the vapors may be irritating to the eyes.

Herbal Compresses

Herbs may be applied directly to an area to promote a healing effect, such as to the chest for relieving congestion or alleviating a spasmodic cough. You will need a piece of flannel, large enough to be doubled across the area to be treated (usually the chest); a clean, dry towel; and a hot infusion. To begin, prepare 2 cups of an infusion (following the instructions on page 24) using 2 teaspoons of freshly grated gingerroot or 2 tablespoons of peppermint leaf. Soak the flannel in the infusion, which should be comfortably hot. Wring out and place on the bare chest. Cover with a dry towel. To prolong the heating effects, place a hot-water bottle on top.

A COMPRESS FOR THE FEET:
THE WARMING SOCKS TREATMENT

Thin cotton socks
Chilled infusion of garlic, gingerroot, catnip, or peppermint
Wool socks

Thoroughly drench the cotton socks in the prepared infusion. Wring out well and place on prewarmed feet. Immediately put on the wool socks and go to bed. The cold socks will have a dual action: They draw congestion from the head and stimulate the body's immune system. The socks will dry in a couple of hours but may be left on all night.

Caution: Do not use this if the patient is very chilled or debilitated.

A WHOLE-BODY COMPRESS TO REDUCE FEVER

This treatment is especially useful in resolving fevers and relieving pain and spasm. The sheet will first cool you, then warm you, then encourage perspiration, and finally return you to a comfortable, neutral temperature. It's also very relaxing and may induce a long, deep sleep.

2 wool blankets
A clean sheet
1 quart chilled infusion of catnip, gingerroot, lemon balm,
  or peppermint

Place the wool blankets across a bed. Thoroughly saturate the sheet in the infusion and wring it out. Place the sheet on top of the wool blankets on the bed. Lie down on the sheet, naked, and wrap the sheet and blankets around you.

While the sheet will be very cold at first, your body heat will soon warm it up. If you are very chilled, you may place a hot-water bottle at your feet and put on a wool cap.

Children respond very well to a shortened version of this treatment. Keep them in the sheet only until it is warm and/or dry. Although they may initially fuss from the cold sheet, the reduction in fever will soon make them comfortable and content.

CONVERTING RECIPE MEASUREMENTS TO METRIC

Use the following chart for converting U.S. measurements to metric. Since these conversions are not exact, it's important to convert the measurements for all of the ingredients to maintain the proportions of the original recipe.

To convert to	From	Multiply by
milliliters	teaspoons	4.93
milliliters	tablespoons	14.79
milliliters	fluid ounces	29.57
milliliters	cups	236.59
liters	cups	0.236
grams	ounces	28.35

Resources

Use your local health food or natural grocery store as a resource for vitamins and herbs. If you can't find what you need locally, the following suppliers may be able to help.

Herb Suppliers

Avena Botanicals
(866) 282-8362
www.avenabotanicals.com

Blessed Herbs
(800) 489-4372
www.blessedherbs.com

Frontier Cooperative Herbs
(844) 550-6200
www.frontiercoop.com

Herb Pharm
(800) 348-4372
www.herb-pharm.com

Sage Mountain Botanical
Sanctuary
https://sagemountain.com

Wise Woman Herbals
541-895-5152
https://wisewomanherbals.com

Supplement Suppliers

Energique Inc.
(800) 869-8078
www.energiquepro.com
This supplier carries a wide variety of herbs and nutritional supplements.

New Chapter
(800) 543-7279
www.newchapter.com
New Chapter also makes a wonderful ginger syrup you can use to create cough and flu formulas.

Pioneer Nutritional Formulas
(800) 660-7742
https://pioneernutritional.com
Many of Pioneer's products combine vitamins with synergistic herbs.

Rainbow Light
(800) 475-1890
www.rainbowlight.com
Rainbow Light formulates vegetarian supplements.

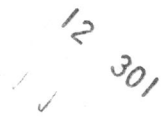